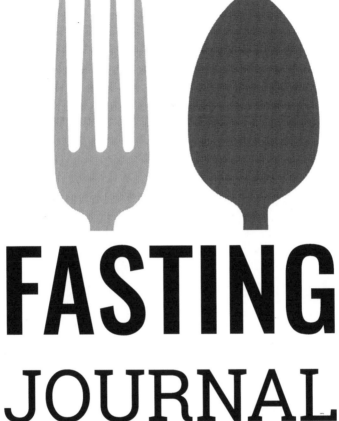

FASTING

JOURNAL

GOALS

Date					
	Goal	Day 1	Day 30	Day 60	Day 90 !
Weight					
Chest					
Waist					
Hips					
Thighs					
Arms					

Other Goals (energy level, cravings, digestion, skin ....)

HOURS FASTED BEFORE EATING: _____

HUNGER LEVEL:
1 2 3 4 5 6 7 8 9 10

M T W T F S S

DATE: _____

WEIGHT: _____

DAY 1

Time	Food/Beverage	Calories

STARTED NEW FAST AT: _____ / NA   ENERGY LEVEL: 1 2 3 4 5 6 7 8 9 10

CHECK NUMBER OF 8 OZ
GLASSES OF WATER: ☐ ☐ ☐ ☐ ☐ ☐ ☐ ☐ ☐ ☐

Time	Exercise	Amount

MOOD/CHALLENGES/NSV'S:

_____

_____

_____

DAY 2	M T W T F S S DATE: _____ WEIGHT: _____	HOURS FASTED BEFORE EATING: _____ HUNGER LEVEL: 1 2 3 4 5 6 7 8 9 10

Time	Food/Beverage	Calories

STARTED NEW FAST AT: _____/ NA   ENERGY LEVEL: 1 2 3 4 5 6 7 8 9 10

CHECK NUMBER OF 8 OZ
GLASSES OF WATER:

Time	Exercise	Amount

MOOD/CHALLENGES/NSV'S:
_____
_____
_____
_____

HOURS FASTED BEFORE EATING: _____

HUNGER LEVEL:

1 2 3 4 5 6 7 8 9 10

M T W T F S S

DATE: _____

WEIGHT: _____

DAY 3

Time	Food/Beverage	Calories

STARTED NEW FAST AT: _____ / NA   ENERGY LEVEL: 1 2 3 4 5 6 7 8 9 10

CHECK NUMBER OF 8 OZ GLASSES OF WATER:

Time	Exercise	Amount

MOOD/CHALLENGES/NSV'S:

_____

_____

_____

DAY 4

M T W T F S S

DATE: _____

WEIGHT: _____

HOURS FASTED BEFORE EATING: _____

HUNGER LEVEL:
1 2 3 4 5 6 7 8 9 10

Time	Food/Beverage	Calories

STARTED NEW FAST AT: _____ / NA   ENERGY LEVEL: 1 2 3 4 5 6 7 8 9 10

CHECK NUMBER OF 8 OZ
GLASSES OF WATER:

Time	Exercise	Amount

MOOD/CHALLENGES/NSV'S:

_____

_____

_____

_____

HOURS FASTED BEFORE EATING: _____

HUNGER LEVEL:
1 2 3 4 5 6 7 8 9 10

M T W T F S S

DATE: _____

WEIGHT: _____

Time	Food/Beverage	Calories

STARTED NEW FAST AT: _____ / NA   ENERGY LEVEL: 1 2 3 4 5 6 7 8 9 10

CHECK NUMBER OF 8 OZ
GLASSES OF WATER:

Time	Exercise	Amount

MOOD/CHALLENGES/NSV'S: _____

_____

_____

_____

DAY 6

M T W T F S S

DATE: _____

WEIGHT: _____

HOURS FASTED BEFORE EATING: _____

HUNGER LEVEL:
1 2 3 4 5 6 7 8 9 10

Time	Food/Beverage	Calories

STARTED NEW FAST AT: _____ / NA   ENERGY LEVEL: 1 2 3 4 5 6 7 8 9 10

CHECK NUMBER OF 8 OZ GLASSES OF WATER:

Time	Exercise	Amount

MOOD/CHALLENGES/NSV'S:

_____

_____

_____

_____

HOURS FASTED BEFORE EATING: _____

HUNGER LEVEL:
1 2 3 4 5 6 7 8 9 10

M T W T F S S

DATE: _____

WEIGHT: _____

DAY 7

Time	Food/Beverage	Calories

STARTED NEW FAST AT: _____ / NA   ENERGY LEVEL: 1 2 3 4 5 6 7 8 9 10

CHECK NUMBER OF 8 OZ
GLASSES OF WATER: ☐ ☐ ☐ ☐ ☐ ☐ ☐ ☐ ☐ ☐

Time	Exercise	Amount

MOOD/CHALLENGES/NSV'S:

_____

_____

_____

DAY 8

M T W T F S S

DATE: _____

WEIGHT: _____

HOURS FASTED BEFORE EATING: _____

HUNGER LEVEL:
1 2 3 4 5 6 7 8 9 10

Time	Food/Beverage	Calories

STARTED NEW FAST AT: _____ / NA   ENERGY LEVEL: 1 2 3 4 5 6 7 8 9 10

CHECK NUMBER OF 8 OZ
GLASSES OF WATER:

Time	Exercise	Amount

MOOD/CHALLENGES/NSV'S:
_____
_____
_____
_____

HOURS FASTED BEFORE EATING: _____

HUNGER LEVEL:
1 2 3 4 5 6 7 8 9 10

M T W T F S S

DATE: _____

WEIGHT: _____

DAY
9

Time	Food/Beverage	Calories

STARTED NEW FAST AT: _____ / NA   ENERGY LEVEL: 1 2 3 4 5 6 7 8 9 10

CHECK NUMBER OF 8 OZ
GLASSES OF WATER:

Time	Exercise	Amount

MOOD/CHALLENGES/NSV'S: _____
_____
_____
_____

DAY 10

M T W T F S S

DATE: _____

WEIGHT: _____

HOURS FASTED BEFORE EATING: _____

HUNGER LEVEL:
1 2 3 4 5 6 7 8 9 10

Time	Food/Beverage	Calories

STARTED NEW FAST AT: _____ / NA   ENERGY LEVEL: 1 2 3 4 5 6 7 8 9 10

CHECK NUMBER OF 8 OZ GLASSES OF WATER:

Time	Exercise	Amount

MOOD/CHALLENGES/NSV'S:

_____

_____

_____

_____

HOURS FASTED BEFORE EATING: _____

HUNGER LEVEL:
1 2 3 4 5 6 7 8 9 10

M T W T F S S

DATE: _____

WEIGHT: _____

DAY
11

Time	Food/Beverage	Calories

STARTED NEW FAST AT: _____ / NA   ENERGY LEVEL: 1 2 3 4 5 6 7 8 9 10

CHECK NUMBER OF 8 OZ
GLASSES OF WATER:

Time	Exercise	Amount

MOOD/CHALLENGES/NSV'S: _____
_____
_____
_____

M T W T F S S

DATE: _____

WEIGHT: _____

HOURS FASTED BEFORE EATING: _____

HUNGER LEVEL:
1 2 3 4 5 6 7 8 9 10

Time	Food/Beverage	Calories

STARTED NEW FAST AT: _____ / NA   ENERGY LEVEL: 1 2 3 4 5 6 7 8 9 10

CHECK NUMBER OF 8 OZ
GLASSES OF WATER:

Time	Exercise	Amount

MOOD/CHALLENGES/NSV'S:
_____
_____
_____
_____

HOURS FASTED BEFORE EATING: _____

HUNGER LEVEL:
1 2 3 4 5 6 7 8 9 10

M T W T F S S

DATE: _____

WEIGHT: _____

DAY 13

Time	Food/Beverage	Calories

STARTED NEW FAST AT: _____ / NA   ENERGY LEVEL: 1 2 3 4 5 6 7 8 9 10

CHECK NUMBER OF 8 OZ
GLASSES OF WATER:

Time	Exercise	Amount

MOOD/CHALLENGES/NSV'S:

DAY 14

M T W T F S S

DATE: _____

WEIGHT: _____

HOURS FASTED BEFORE EATING: _____

HUNGER LEVEL:
1 2 3 4 5 6 7 8 9 10

Time	Food/Beverage	Calories

STARTED NEW FAST AT: _____ / NA   ENERGY LEVEL: 1 2 3 4 5 6 7 8 9 10

CHECK NUMBER OF 8 OZ
GLASSES OF WATER:

Time	Exercise	Amount

MOOD/CHALLENGES/NSV'S: _____

_____

_____

HOURS FASTED BEFORE EATING: _____	M T W T F S S	DAY
HUNGER LEVEL:	DATE: _____	15
1 2 3 4 5 6 7 8 9 10	WEIGHT: _____	

Time	Food/Beverage	Calories

STARTED NEW FAST AT: _____ / NA   ENERGY LEVEL: 1 2 3 4 5 6 7 8 9 10

CHECK NUMBER OF 8 OZ GLASSES OF WATER:

Time	Exercise	Amount

MOOD/CHALLENGES/NSV'S:

_____

_____

_____

DAY 16

M T W T F S S

DATE: _____

WEIGHT: _____

HOURS FASTED BEFORE EATING: _____

HUNGER LEVEL:
1 2 3 4 5 6 7 8 9 10

Time	Food/Beverage	Calories

STARTED NEW FAST AT: _____ / NA   ENERGY LEVEL: 1 2 3 4 5 6 7 8 9 10

CHECK NUMBER OF 8 OZ GLASSES OF WATER:

Time	Exercise	Amount

MOOD/CHALLENGES/NSV'S: _____
_____
_____
_____

HOURS FASTED BEFORE EATING: _____

HUNGER LEVEL:
1 2 3 4 5 6 7 8 9 10

M T W T F S S

DATE: _____

WEIGHT: _____

DAY 17

Time	Food/Beverage	Calories

STARTED NEW FAST AT: _____ / NA   ENERGY LEVEL: 1 2 3 4 5 6 7 8 9 10

CHECK NUMBER OF 8 OZ
GLASSES OF WATER:

Time	Exercise	Amount

MOOD/CHALLENGES/NSV'S:

_____

_____

_____

DAY 18	M T W T F S S DATE: _____ WEIGHT: _____	HOURS FASTED BEFORE EATING: _____ HUNGER LEVEL: 1 2 3 4 5 6 7 8 9 10

Time	Food/Beverage	Calories

STARTED NEW FAST AT: _____ / NA   ENERGY LEVEL: 1 2 3 4 5 6 7 8 9 10

CHECK NUMBER OF 8 OZ GLASSES OF WATER:

Time	Exercise	Amount

MOOD/CHALLENGES/NSV'S:

_____

_____

_____

_____

HOURS FASTED BEFORE EATING: _____

HUNGER LEVEL:
1 2 3 4 5 6 7 8 9 10

M T W T F S S

DATE: _____

WEIGHT: _____

Time	Food/Beverage	Calories

STARTED NEW FAST AT: _____ / NA   ENERGY LEVEL: 1 2 3 4 5 6 7 8 9 10

CHECK NUMBER OF 8 OZ
GLASSES OF WATER:

Time	Exercise	Amount

MOOD/CHALLENGES/NSV'S:
_____
_____
_____
_____

DAY 20	M T W T F S S DATE: _____ WEIGHT: _____	HOURS FASTED BEFORE EATING: _____ HUNGER LEVEL: 1 2 3 4 5 6 7 8 9 10

Time	Food/Beverage	Calories

STARTED NEW FAST AT: _____ / NA   ENERGY LEVEL: 1 2 3 4 5 6 7 8 9 10

CHECK NUMBER OF 8 OZ GLASSES OF WATER:

Time	Exercise	Amount

MOOD/CHALLENGES/NSV'S:

_____

_____

_____

_____

HOURS FASTED BEFORE EATING: _____

HUNGER LEVEL:
1 2 3 4 5 6 7 8 9 10

M T W T F S S

DATE: _____

WEIGHT: _____

DAY 21

Time	Food/Beverage	Calories

STARTED NEW FAST AT: _____ / NA   ENERGY LEVEL: 1 2 3 4 5 6 7 8 9 10

CHECK NUMBER OF 8 OZ
GLASSES OF WATER:

Time	Exercise	Amount

MOOD/CHALLENGES/NSV'S:
_____
_____
_____
_____

DAY 22

M T W T F S S

DATE: _____

WEIGHT: _____

HOURS FASTED BEFORE EATING: _____

HUNGER LEVEL:
1 2 3 4 5 6 7 8 9 10

Time	Food/Beverage	Calories

STARTED NEW FAST AT: _____ / NA   ENERGY LEVEL: 1 2 3 4 5 6 7 8 9 10

CHECK NUMBER OF 8 OZ
GLASSES OF WATER:

Time	Exercise	Amount

MOOD/CHALLENGES/NSV'S: _____

_____

_____

_____

HOURS FASTED BEFORE EATING: _____

HUNGER LEVEL:
1 2 3 4 5 6 7 8 9 10

M T W T F S S

DATE: _____

WEIGHT: _____

DAY
23

Time	Food/Beverage	Calories

STARTED NEW FAST AT: _____ / NA   ENERGY LEVEL: 1 2 3 4 5 6 7 8 9 10

CHECK NUMBER OF 8 OZ
GLASSES OF WATER:

Time	Exercise	Amount

MOOD/CHALLENGES/NSV'S:

_____

_____

_____

DAY 24

M T W T F S S

DATE: _____

WEIGHT: _____

HOURS FASTED BEFORE EATING: _____

HUNGER LEVEL:
1 2 3 4 5 6 7 8 9 10

Time	Food/Beverage	Calories

STARTED NEW FAST AT: _____ / NA   ENERGY LEVEL: 1 2 3 4 5 6 7 8 9 10

CHECK NUMBER OF 8 OZ GLASSES OF WATER:

Time	Exercise	Amount

MOOD/CHALLENGES/NSV'S:
_____
_____
_____
_____

HOURS FASTED BEFORE EATING: _____

HUNGER LEVEL:
1 2 3 4 5 6 7 8 9 10

M T W T F S S

DATE: _____

WEIGHT: _____

DAY 25

Time	Food/Beverage	Calories

STARTED NEW FAST AT: _____ / NA   ENERGY LEVEL: 1 2 3 4 5 6 7 8 9 10

CHECK NUMBER OF 8 OZ GLASSES OF WATER:

Time	Exercise	Amount

MOOD/CHALLENGES/NSV'S: _____
_____
_____
_____

DAY 26	M T W T F S S DATE: _____ WEIGHT: _____	HOURS FASTED BEFORE EATING: _____ HUNGER LEVEL: 1 2 3 4 5 6 7 8 9 10

Time	Food/Beverage	Calories

STARTED NEW FAST AT: _____ / NA   ENERGY LEVEL: 1 2 3 4 5 6 7 8 9 10

CHECK NUMBER OF 8 OZ GLASSES OF WATER:

Time	Exercise	Amount

MOOD/CHALLENGES/NSV'S: _____
_____
_____
_____

HOURS FASTED BEFORE EATING: _____

HUNGER LEVEL:
1 2 3 4 5 6 7 8 9 10

M T W T F S S

DATE: _____

WEIGHT: _____

DAY 27

Time	Food/Beverage	Calories

STARTED NEW FAST AT: _____ / NA   ENERGY LEVEL: 1 2 3 4 5 6 7 8 9 10

CHECK NUMBER OF 8 OZ GLASSES OF WATER:

Time	Exercise	Amount

MOOD/CHALLENGES/NSV'S:
_____
_____
_____
_____

M T W T F S S

DATE: _____

WEIGHT: _____

HOURS FASTED BEFORE EATING: _____

HUNGER LEVEL:
1 2 3 4 5 6 7 8 9 10

Time	Food/Beverage	Calories

STARTED NEW FAST AT: _____ / NA   ENERGY LEVEL: 1 2 3 4 5 6 7 8 9 10

CHECK NUMBER OF 8 OZ GLASSES OF WATER:

Time	Exercise	Amount

MOOD/CHALLENGES/NSV'S: _____

_____

_____

_____

HOURS FASTED BEFORE EATING: _____

HUNGER LEVEL:

1 2 3 4 5 6 7 8 9 10

M T W T F S S

DATE: _____

WEIGHT: _____

DAY
29

Time	Food/Beverage	Calories

STARTED NEW FAST AT: _____ / NA   ENERGY LEVEL: 1 2 3 4 5 6 7 8 9 10

CHECK NUMBER OF 8 OZ
GLASSES OF WATER:

Time	Exercise	Amount

MOOD/CHALLENGES/NSV'S: _____

_____

_____

_____

M T W T F S S

DATE: _____

WEIGHT: _____

HOURS FASTED BEFORE EATING: _____

HUNGER LEVEL:
1 2 3 4 5 6 7 8 9 10

Time	Food/Beverage	Calories

STARTED NEW FAST AT: _____ / NA   ENERGY LEVEL: 1 2 3 4 5 6 7 8 9 10

CHECK NUMBER OF 8 OZ
GLASSES OF WATER:

Time	Exercise	Amount

MOOD/CHALLENGES/NSV'S: _____

_____

_____

_____

HOURS FASTED BEFORE EATING: _____

HUNGER LEVEL:
1 2 3 4 5 6 7 8 9 10

M T W T F S S

DATE: _____

WEIGHT: _____

DAY 31

Time	Food/Beverage	Calories

STARTED NEW FAST AT: _____ / NA   ENERGY LEVEL: 1 2 3 4 5 6 7 8 9 10

CHECK NUMBER OF 8 OZ
GLASSES OF WATER:

Time	Exercise	Amount

MOOD/CHALLENGES/NSV'S: _____

_____

_____

_____

DAY 32	M T W T F S S DATE: _____ WEIGHT: _____	HOURS FASTED BEFORE EATING: _____ HUNGER LEVEL: 1 2 3 4 5 6 7 8 9 10

Time	Food/Beverage	Calories

STARTED NEW FAST AT: _____ / NA   ENERGY LEVEL: 1 2 3 4 5 6 7 8 9 10

CHECK NUMBER OF 8 OZ
GLASSES OF WATER:

Time	Exercise	Amount

MOOD/CHALLENGES/NSV'S: _____

_____

_____

HOURS FASTED BEFORE EATING: _____

HUNGER LEVEL:

1 2 3 4 5 6 7 8 9 10

M T W T F S S

DATE: _____

WEIGHT: _____

DAY 33

Time	Food/Beverage	Calories

STARTED NEW FAST AT: _____ / NA   ENERGY LEVEL: 1 2 3 4 5 6 7 8 9 10

CHECK NUMBER OF 8 OZ
GLASSES OF WATER:

Time	Exercise	Amount

MOOD/CHALLENGES/NSV'S:

_____

_____

_____

DAY 34

M T W T F S S

DATE: _____

WEIGHT: _____

HOURS FASTED BEFORE EATING: _____

HUNGER LEVEL:
1 2 3 4 5 6 7 8 9 10

Time	Food/Beverage	Calories

STARTED NEW FAST AT: _____ / NA   ENERGY LEVEL: 1 2 3 4 5 6 7 8 9 10

CHECK NUMBER OF 8 OZ
GLASSES OF WATER:

Time	Exercise	Amount

MOOD/CHALLENGES/NSV'S: _____

_____

_____

_____

HOURS FASTED BEFORE EATING: _____

HUNGER LEVEL:
1 2 3 4 5 6 7 8 9 10

M T W T F S S

DATE: _____

WEIGHT: _____

DAY
35

Time	Food/Beverage	Calories

STARTED NEW FAST AT: _____ / NA   ENERGY LEVEL: 1 2 3 4 5 6 7 8 9 10

CHECK NUMBER OF 8 OZ
GLASSES OF WATER:

Time	Exercise	Amount

MOOD/CHALLENGES/NSV'S: _____
_____
_____
_____

DAY 36

M T W T F S S

DATE: _____

WEIGHT: _____

HOURS FASTED BEFORE EATING: _____

HUNGER LEVEL:
1 2 3 4 5 6 7 8 9 10

Time	Food/Beverage	Calories

STARTED NEW FAST AT: _____/ NA   ENERGY LEVEL: 1 2 3 4 5 6 7 8 9 10

CHECK NUMBER OF 8 OZ GLASSES OF WATER:

Time	Exercise	Amount

MOOD/CHALLENGES/NSV'S:

_____

_____

_____

	HOURS FASTED BEFORE EATING: _____	M T W T F S S	DAY
	HUNGER LEVEL:	DATE: _____	37
	1 2 3 4 5 6 7 8 9 10	WEIGHT: _____	

Time	Food/Beverage	Calories

STARTED NEW FAST AT: _____ / NA   ENERGY LEVEL: 1 2 3 4 5 6 7 8 9 10

CHECK NUMBER OF 8 OZ
GLASSES OF WATER:

Time	Exercise	Amount

MOOD/CHALLENGES/NSV'S:

_____

_____

_____

DAY 38

M T W T F S S

DATE: _____

WEIGHT: _____

Time	Food/Beverage	Calories

STARTED NEW FAST AT: _____ / NA   ENERGY LEVEL: 1 2 3 4 5 6 7 8 9 10

CHECK NUMBER OF 8 OZ
GLASSES OF WATER:

Time	Exercise	Amount

MOOD/CHALLENGES/NSV'S: _____

_____

_____

_____

HOURS FASTED BEFORE EATING: _____

HUNGER LEVEL:
1 2 3 4 5 6 7 8 9 10

M T W T F S S

DATE: _____

WEIGHT: _____

DAY
39

Time	Food/Beverage	Calories

STARTED NEW FAST AT: _____/ NA   ENERGY LEVEL: 1 2 3 4 5 6 7 8 9 10

CHECK NUMBER OF 8 OZ
GLASSES OF WATER:

Time	Exercise	Amount

MOOD/CHALLENGES/NSV'S: _____

_____

_____

_____

DAY 40

M T W T F S S

DATE: _____

WEIGHT: _____

Time	Food/Beverage	Calories

STARTED NEW FAST AT: _____/ NA   ENERGY LEVEL: 1 2 3 4 5 6 7 8 9 10

CHECK NUMBER OF 8 OZ
GLASSES OF WATER:

Time	Exercise	Amount

MOOD/CHALLENGES/NSV'S: _____

_____

_____

HOURS FASTED BEFORE EATING: _____

HUNGER LEVEL:
1 2 3 4 5 6 7 8 9 10

M T W T F S S

DATE: _____

WEIGHT: _____

DAY 41

Time	Food/Beverage	Calories

STARTED NEW FAST AT: _____ / NA   ENERGY LEVEL: 1 2 3 4 5 6 7 8 9 10

CHECK NUMBER OF 8 OZ GLASSES OF WATER:

Time	Exercise	Amount

MOOD/CHALLENGES/NSV'S:

_____

_____

_____

M T W T F S S

DATE: _____

WEIGHT: _____

HOURS FASTED BEFORE EATING: _____

HUNGER LEVEL:
1 2 3 4 5 6 7 8 9 10

Time	Food/Beverage	Calories

STARTED NEW FAST AT: _____ / NA   ENERGY LEVEL: 1 2 3 4 5 6 7 8 9 10

CHECK NUMBER OF 8 OZ
GLASSES OF WATER:

Time	Exercise	Amount

MOOD/CHALLENGES/NSV'S: _____

_____

_____

_____

HOURS FASTED BEFORE EATING: _____

HUNGER LEVEL:
1 2 3 4 5 6 7 8 9 10

M T W T F S S

DATE: _____

WEIGHT: _____

DAY 43

Time	Food/Beverage	Calories

STARTED NEW FAST AT: _____ / NA   ENERGY LEVEL: 1 2 3 4 5 6 7 8 9 10

CHECK NUMBER OF 8 OZ
GLASSES OF WATER:

Time	Exercise	Amount

MOOD/CHALLENGES/NSV'S: _____

_____

_____

_____

<table>
<tr><td colspan="2">DAY 44</td><td>M T W T F S S
DATE: _____
WEIGHT: _____</td><td colspan="2">HOURS FASTED BEFORE EATING: _____
HUNGER LEVEL:
1 2 3 4 5 6 7 8 9 10</td></tr>
</table>

Time	Food/Beverage	Calories

STARTED NEW FAST AT: _____ / NA   ENERGY LEVEL: 1 2 3 4 5 6 7 8 9 10

CHECK NUMBER OF 8 OZ GLASSES OF WATER:

Time	Exercise	Amount

MOOD/CHALLENGES/NSV'S: _____

_____

_____

HOURS FASTED BEFORE EATING: _____

HUNGER LEVEL:

1 2 3 4 5 6 7 8 9 10

M T W T F S S

DATE: _____

WEIGHT: _____

Time	Food/Beverage	Calories

STARTED NEW FAST AT: _____/ NA   ENERGY LEVEL: 1 2 3 4 5 6 7 8 9 10

CHECK NUMBER OF 8 OZ
GLASSES OF WATER:

Time	Exercise	Amount

MOOD/CHALLENGES/NSV'S: _____

_____

_____

_____

DAY 46

M T W T F S S

DATE: _____

WEIGHT: _____

HOURS FASTED BEFORE EATING: _____

HUNGER LEVEL:
1 2 3 4 5 6 7 8 9 10

Time	Food/Beverage	Calories

STARTED NEW FAST AT: _____ / NA   ENERGY LEVEL: 1 2 3 4 5 6 7 8 9 10

CHECK NUMBER OF 8 OZ
GLASSES OF WATER:

Time	Exercise	Amount

MOOD/CHALLENGES/NSV'S: _____

_____

_____

_____

HOURS FASTED BEFORE EATING: _____

HUNGER LEVEL:
1 2 3 4 5 6 7 8 9 10

M T W T F S S

DATE: _____

WEIGHT: _____

DAY 47

Time	Food/Beverage	Calories

STARTED NEW FAST AT: _____ / NA   ENERGY LEVEL: 1 2 3 4 5 6 7 8 9 10

CHECK NUMBER OF 8 OZ GLASSES OF WATER:

Time	Exercise	Amount

MOOD/CHALLENGES/NSV'S: _____

_____

_____

_____

DAY 48

M T W T F S S

DATE: _____

WEIGHT: _____

HOURS FASTED BEFORE EATING: _____

HUNGER LEVEL:
1 2 3 4 5 6 7 8 9 10

Time	Food/Beverage	Calories

STARTED NEW FAST AT: _____ / NA   ENERGY LEVEL: 1 2 3 4 5 6 7 8 9 10

CHECK NUMBER OF 8 OZ
GLASSES OF WATER:

Time	Exercise	Amount

MOOD/CHALLENGES/NSV'S: _____

_____

_____

_____

HOURS FASTED BEFORE EATING: _____

HUNGER LEVEL:
1 2 3 4 5 6 7 8 9 10

M T W T F S S

DATE: _____

WEIGHT: _____

DAY 49

Time	Food/Beverage	Calories

STARTED NEW FAST AT: _____/ NA   ENERGY LEVEL: 1 2 3 4 5 6 7 8 9 10

CHECK NUMBER OF 8 OZ GLASSES OF WATER:

Time	Exercise	Amount

MOOD/CHALLENGES/NSV'S: _____

_____

_____

_____

DAY 50	M T W T F S S Date: _____ Weight: _____	Hours fasted before eating: _____ Hunger Level: 1 2 3 4 5 6 7 8 9 10

Time	Food/Beverage	Calories

STARTED NEW FAST AT: _____ / NA   ENERGY LEVEL: 1 2 3 4 5 6 7 8 9 10

CHECK NUMBER OF 8 OZ GLASSES OF WATER:

Time	Exercise	Amount

MOOD/CHALLENGES/NSV'S:
_____
_____
_____
_____

HOURS FASTED BEFORE EATING: _____

HUNGER LEVEL:

1 2 3 4 5 6 7 8 9 10

M T W T F S S

DATE: _____

WEIGHT: _____

Time	Food/Beverage	Calories

STARTED NEW FAST AT: _____/ NA   ENERGY LEVEL: 1 2 3 4 5 6 7 8 9 10

CHECK NUMBER OF 8 OZ
GLASSES OF WATER:

Time	Exercise	Amount

MOOD/CHALLENGES/NSV'S:

_____

_____

_____

DAY 52

M T W T F S S

DATE: _____

WEIGHT: _____

HOURS FASTED BEFORE EATING: _____

HUNGER LEVEL:
1 2 3 4 5 6 7 8 9 10

Time	Food/Beverage	Calories

STARTED NEW FAST AT: _____ / NA   ENERGY LEVEL: 1 2 3 4 5 6 7 8 9 10

CHECK NUMBER OF 8 OZ GLASSES OF WATER:

Time	Exercise	Amount

MOOD/CHALLENGES/NSV'S: _____
_____
_____
_____

HOURS FASTED BEFORE EATING: _____

HUNGER LEVEL:
1 2 3 4 5 6 7 8 9 10

M T W T F S S

DATE: _____

WEIGHT: _____

Time	Food/Beverage	Calories

STARTED NEW FAST AT: _____/ NA   ENERGY LEVEL: 1 2 3 4 5 6 7 8 9 10

CHECK NUMBER OF 8 OZ
GLASSES OF WATER:

Time	Exercise	Amount

MOOD/CHALLENGES/NSV'S:

_____

_____

_____

DAY 54

M T W T F S S

DATE: _____

WEIGHT: _____

HOURS FASTED BEFORE EATING: _____

HUNGER LEVEL:
1 2 3 4 5 6 7 8 9 10

Time	Food/Beverage	Calories

STARTED NEW FAST AT: _____ / NA   ENERGY LEVEL: 1 2 3 4 5 6 7 8 9 10

CHECK NUMBER OF 8 OZ
GLASSES OF WATER:

Time	Exercise	Amount

MOOD/CHALLENGES/NSV'S: _____

_____

_____

_____

HOURS FASTED BEFORE EATING: _____

HUNGER LEVEL:
1 2 3 4 5 6 7 8 9 10

M T W T F S S

DATE: _____

WEIGHT: _____

DAY
55

Time	Food/Beverage	Calories

STARTED NEW FAST AT: _____ / NA   ENERGY LEVEL: 1 2 3 4 5 6 7 8 9 10

CHECK NUMBER OF 8 OZ
GLASSES OF WATER:

Time	Exercise	Amount

MOOD/CHALLENGES/NSV'S:

_____

_____

_____

DAY 56

M T W T F S S

DATE: _____

WEIGHT: _____

HOURS FASTED BEFORE EATING: _____

HUNGER LEVEL:
1 2 3 4 5 6 7 8 9 10

Time	Food/Beverage	Calories

STARTED NEW FAST AT: _____ / NA   ENERGY LEVEL: 1 2 3 4 5 6 7 8 9 10

CHECK NUMBER OF 8 OZ
GLASSES OF WATER:

Time	Exercise	Amount

MOOD/CHALLENGES/NSV'S: _____

_____

_____

_____

HOURS FASTED BEFORE EATING: _____

HUNGER LEVEL:
1 2 3 4 5 6 7 8 9 10

M T W T F S S

DATE: _____

WEIGHT: _____

DAY 57

Time	Food/Beverage	Calories

STARTED NEW FAST AT: _____ / NA   ENERGY LEVEL: 1 2 3 4 5 6 7 8 9 10

CHECK NUMBER OF 8 OZ GLASSES OF WATER:

Time	Exercise	Amount

MOOD/CHALLENGES/NSV'S:
_____

_____

_____

M T W T F S S

DATE: _____

WEIGHT: _____

HOURS FASTED BEFORE EATING: _____

HUNGER LEVEL:
1 2 3 4 5 6 7 8 9 10

Time	Food/Beverage	Calories

STARTED NEW FAST AT: _____ / NA   ENERGY LEVEL: 1 2 3 4 5 6 7 8 9 10

CHECK NUMBER OF 8 OZ GLASSES OF WATER:

Time	Exercise	Amount

MOOD/CHALLENGES/NSV'S: _____

_____

_____

HOURS FASTED BEFORE EATING: _____

HUNGER LEVEL:
1 2 3 4 5 6 7 8 9 10

M T W T F S S

DATE: _____

WEIGHT: _____

DAY 59

Time	Food/Beverage	Calories

STARTED NEW FAST AT: _____ / NA   ENERGY LEVEL: 1 2 3 4 5 6 7 8 9 10

CHECK NUMBER OF 8 OZ GLASSES OF WATER:

Time	Exercise	Amount

MOOD/CHALLENGES/NSV'S:
_____
_____
_____

DAY 60

M T W T F S S

DATE: _____

WEIGHT: _____

HOURS FASTED BEFORE EATING: _____

HUNGER LEVEL:
1 2 3 4 5 6 7 8 9 10

Time	Food/Beverage	Calories

STARTED NEW FAST AT: _____ / NA   ENERGY LEVEL: 1 2 3 4 5 6 7 8 9 10

CHECK NUMBER OF 8 OZ GLASSES OF WATER:

Time	Exercise	Amount

MOOD/CHALLENGES/NSV'S: _____

_____

_____

_____

HOURS FASTED BEFORE EATING: _____

HUNGER LEVEL:

1 2 3 4 5 6 7 8 9 10

M T W T F S S

DATE: _____

WEIGHT: _____

DAY 61

Time	Food/Beverage	Calories

STARTED NEW FAST AT: _____ / NA   ENERGY LEVEL: 1 2 3 4 5 6 7 8 9 10

CHECK NUMBER OF 8 OZ
GLASSES OF WATER:

Time	Exercise	Amount

MOOD/CHALLENGES/NSV'S:

_____

_____

_____

DAY 62

M T W T F S S

DATE: _____

WEIGHT: _____

HOURS FASTED BEFORE EATING: _____

HUNGER LEVEL:
1 2 3 4 5 6 7 8 9 10

Time	Food/Beverage	Calories

STARTED NEW FAST AT: _____ / NA   ENERGY LEVEL: 1 2 3 4 5 6 7 8 9 10

CHECK NUMBER OF 8 OZ GLASSES OF WATER:

Time	Exercise	Amount

MOOD/CHALLENGES/NSV'S: _____
_____
_____
_____

HOURS FASTED BEFORE EATING: _____

HUNGER LEVEL:
1 2 3 4 5 6 7 8 9 10

M T W T F S S

DATE: _____

WEIGHT: _____

DAY
63

Time	Food/Beverage	Calories

STARTED NEW FAST AT: _____ / NA   ENERGY LEVEL: 1 2 3 4 5 6 7 8 9 10

CHECK NUMBER OF 8 OZ
GLASSES OF WATER:

Time	Exercise	Amount

MOOD/CHALLENGES/NSV'S:
_____
_____
_____

DAY 64	M T W T F S S DATE: _____ WEIGHT: _____	HOURS FASTED BEFORE EATING: _____ HUNGER LEVEL: 1 2 3 4 5 6 7 8 9 10

Time	Food/Beverage	Calories

STARTED NEW FAST AT: _____ / NA   ENERGY LEVEL: 1 2 3 4 5 6 7 8 9 10

CHECK NUMBER OF 8 OZ GLASSES OF WATER:

Time	Exercise	Amount

MOOD/CHALLENGES/NSV'S: _____

_____

_____

_____

HOURS FASTED BEFORE EATING: _____

HUNGER LEVEL:
1 2 3 4 5 6 7 8 9 10

M T W T F S S

DATE: _____

WEIGHT: _____

DAY
65

Time	Food/Beverage	Calories

STARTED NEW FAST AT: _____/ NA   ENERGY LEVEL: 1 2 3 4 5 6 7 8 9 10

CHECK NUMBER OF 8 OZ GLASSES OF WATER:

Time	Exercise	Amount

MOOD/CHALLENGES/NSV'S:
_____

_____

_____

_____

DAY 66	M T W T F S S DATE: _____ WEIGHT: _____	HOURS FASTED BEFORE EATING: _____ HUNGER LEVEL: 1 2 3 4 5 6 7 8 9 10

Time	Food/Beverage	Calories

STARTED NEW FAST AT: _____ / NA   ENERGY LEVEL: 1 2 3 4 5 6 7 8 9 10

CHECK NUMBER OF 8 OZ
GLASSES OF WATER:

Time	Exercise	Amount

MOOD/CHALLENGES/NSV'S: _____

_____

_____

_____

HOURS FASTED BEFORE EATING: _____

HUNGER LEVEL:

1 2 3 4 5 6 7 8 9 10

M T W T F S S

DATE: _____

WEIGHT: _____

DAY 67

Time	Food/Beverage	Calories

STARTED NEW FAST AT: _____/ NA   ENERGY LEVEL: 1 2 3 4 5 6 7 8 9 10

CHECK NUMBER OF 8 OZ GLASSES OF WATER:

Time	Exercise	Amount

MOOD/CHALLENGES/NSV'S:

_____

_____

_____

DAY 68	M T W T F S S DATE: _____ WEIGHT: _____	HOURS FASTED BEFORE EATING: _____ HUNGER LEVEL: 1 2 3 4 5 6 7 8 9 10

Time	Food/Beverage	Calories

STARTED NEW FAST AT: _____ / NA   ENERGY LEVEL: 1 2 3 4 5 6 7 8 9 10

CHECK NUMBER OF 8 OZ
GLASSES OF WATER:

Time	Exercise	Amount

MOOD/CHALLENGES/NSV'S: _____

_____

_____

_____

HOURS FASTED BEFORE EATING: _____

HUNGER LEVEL:
1 2 3 4 5 6 7 8 9 10

M T W T F S S

DATE: _____

WEIGHT: _____

DAY 69

Time	Food/Beverage	Calories

STARTED NEW FAST AT: _____ / NA   ENERGY LEVEL: 1 2 3 4 5 6 7 8 9 10

CHECK NUMBER OF 8 OZ
GLASSES OF WATER:

Time	Exercise	Amount

MOOD/CHALLENGES/NSV'S: _____

_____

_____

_____

M T W T F S S

DATE: _____

WEIGHT: _____

Time	Food/Beverage	Calories

STARTED NEW FAST AT: _____/ NA   ENERGY LEVEL: 1 2 3 4 5 6 7 8 9 10

CHECK NUMBER OF 8 OZ
GLASSES OF WATER:

Time	Exercise	Amount

MOOD/CHALLENGES/NSV'S:
_____
_____
_____
_____

HOURS FASTED BEFORE EATING: _____

HUNGER LEVEL:

1 2 3 4 5 6 7 8 9 10

M T W T F S S

DATE: _____

WEIGHT: _____

DAY 71

Time	Food/Beverage	Calories

STARTED NEW FAST AT: _____ / NA   ENERGY LEVEL: 1 2 3 4 5 6 7 8 9 10

CHECK NUMBER OF 8 OZ GLASSES OF WATER:

Time	Exercise	Amount

MOOD/CHALLENGES/NSV'S: _____

_____

_____

_____

DAY 72

M T W T F S S

DATE: _____

WEIGHT: _____

HOURS FASTED BEFORE EATING: _____

HUNGER LEVEL:
1 2 3 4 5 6 7 8 9 10

Time	Food/Beverage	Calories

STARTED NEW FAST AT: _____/ NA   ENERGY LEVEL: 1 2 3 4 5 6 7 8 9 10

CHECK NUMBER OF 8 OZ GLASSES OF WATER:

Time	Exercise	Amount

MOOD/CHALLENGES/NSV'S: _____
_____
_____
_____

HOURS FASTED BEFORE EATING: _____

HUNGER LEVEL:
1 2 3 4 5 6 7 8 9 10

M T W T F S S

DATE: _____

WEIGHT: _____

DAY 73

Time	Food/Beverage	Calories

STARTED NEW FAST AT: _____ / NA   ENERGY LEVEL: 1 2 3 4 5 6 7 8 9 10

CHECK NUMBER OF 8 OZ GLASSES OF WATER:

Time	Exercise	Amount

MOOD/CHALLENGES/NSV'S:

_____

_____

_____

DAY 74	M T W T F S S DATE: _____ WEIGHT: _____	HOURS FASTED BEFORE EATING: _____ HUNGER LEVEL: 1 2 3 4 5 6 7 8 9 10

Time	Food/Beverage	Calories

STARTED NEW FAST AT: _____ / NA   ENERGY LEVEL: 1 2 3 4 5 6 7 8 9 10

CHECK NUMBER OF 8 OZ
GLASSES OF WATER:

Time	Exercise	Amount

MOOD/CHALLENGES/NSV'S: _____
_____
_____
_____

HOURS FASTED BEFORE EATING: _____

HUNGER LEVEL:

1 2 3 4 5 6 7 8 9 10

M T W T F S S

DATE: _____

WEIGHT: _____

DAY 75

Time	Food/Beverage	Calories

STARTED NEW FAST AT: _____ / NA   ENERGY LEVEL: 1 2 3 4 5 6 7 8 9 10

CHECK NUMBER OF 8 OZ GLASSES OF WATER:

Time	Exercise	Amount

MOOD/CHALLENGES/NSV'S:

_____

_____

_____

DAY 76

M T W T F S S

DATE: _____

WEIGHT: _____

HOURS FASTED BEFORE EATING: _____

HUNGER LEVEL:
1 2 3 4 5 6 7 8 9 10

Time	Food/Beverage	Calories

STARTED NEW FAST AT: _____ / NA   ENERGY LEVEL: 1 2 3 4 5 6 7 8 9 10

CHECK NUMBER OF 8 OZ GLASSES OF WATER:

Time	Exercise	Amount

MOOD/CHALLENGES/NSV'S: _____
_____
_____
_____

HOURS FASTED BEFORE EATING: _____

HUNGER LEVEL:
1 2 3 4 5 6 7 8 9 10

M T W T F S S

DATE: _____

WEIGHT: _____

DAY 77

Time	Food/Beverage	Calories

STARTED NEW FAST AT: _____ / NA   ENERGY LEVEL: 1 2 3 4 5 6 7 8 9 10

CHECK NUMBER OF 8 OZ
GLASSES OF WATER:

Time	Exercise	Amount

MOOD/CHALLENGES/NSV'S:

_____

_____

_____

M T W T F S S

DATE: _____

WEIGHT: _____

HOURS FASTED BEFORE EATING: _____

HUNGER LEVEL:
1 2 3 4 5 6 7 8 9 10

Time	Food/Beverage	Calories

STARTED NEW FAST AT: _____ / NA   ENERGY LEVEL: 1 2 3 4 5 6 7 8 9 10

CHECK NUMBER OF 8 OZ
GLASSES OF WATER:

Time	Exercise	Amount

MOOD/CHALLENGES/NSV'S: _____

_____

_____

_____

HOURS FASTED BEFORE EATING: _____

HUNGER LEVEL:
1 2 3 4 5 6 7 8 9 10

M T W T F S S

DATE: _____

WEIGHT: _____

DAY
79

Time	Food/Beverage	Calories

STARTED NEW FAST AT: _____ / NA   ENERGY LEVEL: 1 2 3 4 5 6 7 8 9 10

CHECK NUMBER OF 8 OZ
GLASSES OF WATER:

Time	Exercise	Amount

MOOD/CHALLENGES/NSV'S:
_____
_____
_____

DAY 80

M T W T F S S

DATE: _____

WEIGHT: _____

HOURS FASTED BEFORE EATING: _____

HUNGER LEVEL:
1 2 3 4 5 6 7 8 9 10

Time	Food/Beverage	Calories

STARTED NEW FAST AT: _____ / NA   ENERGY LEVEL: 1 2 3 4 5 6 7 8 9 10

CHECK NUMBER OF 8 OZ
GLASSES OF WATER:

Time	Exercise	Amount

MOOD/CHALLENGES/NSV'S: _____

_____

_____

_____

HOURS FASTED BEFORE EATING: _____

HUNGER LEVEL:

1 2 3 4 5 6 7 8 9 10

M T W T F S S

DATE: _____

WEIGHT: _____

DAY 81

Time	Food/Beverage	Calories

STARTED NEW FAST AT: _____ / NA   ENERGY LEVEL: 1 2 3 4 5 6 7 8 9 10

CHECK NUMBER OF 8 OZ GLASSES OF WATER:

Time	Exercise	Amount

MOOD/CHALLENGES/NSV'S:

_____

_____

_____

_____

DAY 82

M T W T F S S

DATE: _____

WEIGHT: _____

HOURS FASTED BEFORE EATING: _____

HUNGER LEVEL:
1 2 3 4 5 6 7 8 9 10

Time	Food/Beverage	Calories

STARTED NEW FAST AT: _____ / NA   ENERGY LEVEL: 1 2 3 4 5 6 7 8 9 10

CHECK NUMBER OF 8 OZ GLASSES OF WATER:

Time	Exercise	Amount

MOOD/CHALLENGES/NSV'S: _____

_____

_____

_____

HOURS FASTED BEFORE EATING: _____

HUNGER LEVEL:

1 2 3 4 5 6 7 8 9 10

M T W T F S S

DATE: _____

WEIGHT: _____

DAY 83

Time	Food/Beverage	Calories

STARTED NEW FAST AT: _____ / NA   ENERGY LEVEL: 1 2 3 4 5 6 7 8 9 10

CHECK NUMBER OF 8 OZ GLASSES OF WATER:

Time	Exercise	Amount

MOOD/CHALLENGES/NSV'S:

_____

_____

_____

	DAY 84	M T W T F S S	HOURS FASTED BEFORE EATING: _____

DAY 84

M T W T F S S

DATE: _____

WEIGHT: _____

HOURS FASTED BEFORE EATING: _____

HUNGER LEVEL:
1 2 3 4 5 6 7 8 9 10

Time	Food/Beverage	Calories

STARTED NEW FAST AT: _____ / NA   ENERGY LEVEL: 1 2 3 4 5 6 7 8 9 10

CHECK NUMBER OF 8 OZ GLASSES OF WATER:

Time	Exercise	Amount

MOOD/CHALLENGES/NSV'S: _____

_____

_____

_____

HOURS FASTED BEFORE EATING: _____

HUNGER LEVEL:

1 2 3 4 5 6 7 8 9 10

M T W T F S S

DATE: _____

WEIGHT: _____

DAY
85

Time	Food/Beverage	Calories

STARTED NEW FAST AT: _____ / NA   ENERGY LEVEL: 1 2 3 4 5 6 7 8 9 10

CHECK NUMBER OF 8 OZ
GLASSES OF WATER:

Time	Exercise	Amount

MOOD/CHALLENGES/NSV'S: _____

_____

_____

_____

DAY 86

M T W T F S S

DATE: _____

WEIGHT: _____

HOURS FASTED BEFORE EATING: _____

HUNGER LEVEL:
1 2 3 4 5 6 7 8 9 10

Time	Food/Beverage	Calories

STARTED NEW FAST AT: _____ / NA   ENERGY LEVEL: 1 2 3 4 5 6 7 8 9 10

CHECK NUMBER OF 8 OZ
GLASSES OF WATER:

Time	Exercise	Amount

MOOD/CHALLENGES/NSV'S: _____

_____

_____

_____

HOURS FASTED BEFORE EATING: _____

HUNGER LEVEL:

1 2 3 4 5 6 7 8 9 10

M T W T F S S

DATE: _____

WEIGHT: _____

DAY 87

Time	Food/Beverage	Calories

STARTED NEW FAST AT: _____ / NA   ENERGY LEVEL: 1 2 3 4 5 6 7 8 9 10

CHECK NUMBER OF 8 OZ
GLASSES OF WATER:

Time	Exercise	Amount

MOOD/CHALLENGES/NSV'S:

_____

_____

_____

_____

DAY 88	M T W T F S S DATE: _____ WEIGHT: _____	HOURS FASTED BEFORE EATING: _____ HUNGER LEVEL: 1 2 3 4 5 6 7 8 9 10

Time	Food/Beverage	Calories

STARTED NEW FAST AT: _____ / NA   ENERGY LEVEL: 1 2 3 4 5 6 7 8 9 10

CHECK NUMBER OF 8 OZ
GLASSES OF WATER:

Time	Exercise	Amount

MOOD/CHALLENGES/NSV'S: _____

_____

_____

_____

HOURS FASTED BEFORE EATING: _____

HUNGER LEVEL:
1 2 3 4 5 6 7 8 9 10

M T W T F S S

DATE: _____

WEIGHT: _____

DAY 89

Time	Food/Beverage	Calories

STARTED NEW FAST AT: _____ / NA   ENERGY LEVEL: 1 2 3 4 5 6 7 8 9 10

CHECK NUMBER OF 8 OZ
GLASSES OF WATER:

Time	Exercise	Amount

MOOD/CHALLENGES/NSV'S: _____

_____

_____

_____

DAY 90 !

M T W T F S S

DATE: _____

WEIGHT: _____

HOURS FASTED BEFORE EATING: _____

HUNGER LEVEL:
1 2 3 4 5 6 7 8 9 10

Time	Food/Beverage	Calories

STARTED NEW FAST AT: _____ / NA   ENERGY LEVEL: 1 2 3 4 5 6 7 8 9 10

CHECK NUMBER OF 8 OZ
GLASSES OF WATER:

Time	Exercise	Amount

MOOD/CHALLENGES/NSV'S: _____

_____

_____

_____

Made in the USA
Middletown, DE
24 December 2020